24 HR JUICE FAST

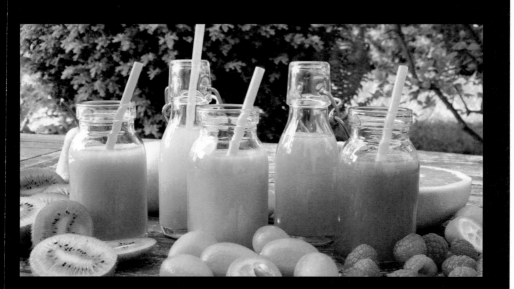

BY: COACH LAWRENCE

* DISCLAIMER *

"The information provided by the health and wellness coach is not intended to be a substitute for professional medical advice, diagnosis, or treatment.
"The health and wellness coach makes no guarantees or promises regarding the results you will achieve from participating in their program or services."

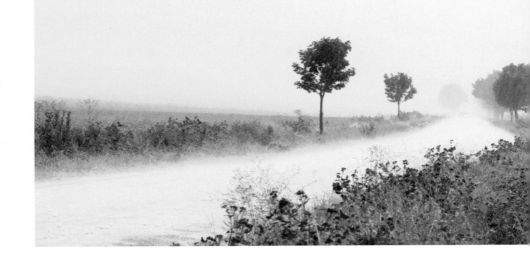

CONTENTS:

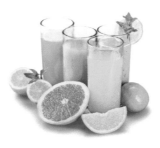

BENEFITS OF FASTING:

When you fast you give your digestive system a break.
This allows more blood to be utilized by your body to begin the detoxifying process. In this phase the body starts removing harmful chemicals. Additional benefits include lowering cholesterol, and blood pressure. Through the process of fasting the lungs, kidneys, and liver. can have the time to replenish themselves.

WHAT IS FASTING?

<u>Fasting</u> - Abstaining from food or drink or both for health, religious, ethical, or ritualistic reasons. Either for short, long, or intermittent periods.

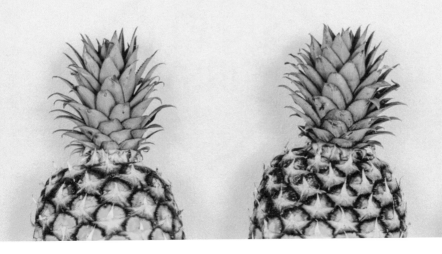

WHO SHOULD NOT FAST:

1. if you are pregnant or nursing.
2. Those with any kind of heart conditions.
3. Anyone with diabetes.

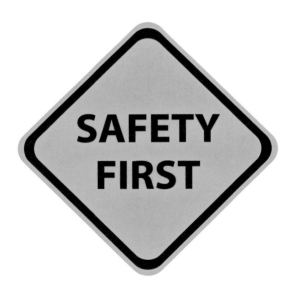

24 HR FASTING PROTOCOL

Possible side effects of fasting; headaches, drowsiness, and hunger pangs.

Juice or water fast?

It is suggested to do a combination of fresh juice and quality water rather than just water alone, as the addition of fresh juices can help nourish the body and shed extra pounds.

* If new to fasting it is recommended to make a vegetable broth to suppress feelings of hunger.

VEGETABLE BROTH RECIPE:

4 cups quality water
1/2 well-scrubbed potato, chopped
1/2 cup grated beets
1/2 cup sliced carrots
1/2 cup chopped celery
1/2 cup sliced onion
2 cloves garlic, minced
1 bay leaf
2 cloves garlic, minced
1 pinch dried thyme
1 pinch powdered cayenne pepper

1. Put all of the ingredients into a pot and bring to a boil over high heat.
2. Lower the heat to a simmering temperature and allow the soup to simmer for one hour
3. Remove from heat and strain out the vegetables (remove bay leaf)
Drink a large glass while fasting. (As much as needed to suppress the feeling of hunger)

One day fast

Upon waking drink one cup of lemon water, either warm or cold. (Room temperature is best for the body to absorb)

* How to prepare

2 quartz of quality water
Juice of 3 lemons
1/2 teaspoon of stevia or blackstrap molasses (optional)

lace the water in a pitcher. Stir in lemon juice and add stevia or molasses. Serve at room temperature

* Two hours later (Example 10:00 am)
Carrot, apple, celery, parsley, beet, and wheatgrass

JUICE RECIPES

CARROT JUICE

Ingredients
6 carrots
1 apple
3 stalks of celery
2 sprigs of parsley
1 beet
a handful of wheatgrass

Directions
Juice the parsley and wheatgrass first. Then, chop the beet in half and the ends off the carrots. Juice the beet first, then the celery, apple, and finish with the carrots. I always like to do carrots at the end as they can sometimes clog the juicer and lower its efficiency.
Grab your favorite glass, pour the juice in (over some ice if you like!), and drink up!

* Two hours later (Example 12- noon) Beetroot, carrot, orange, and spinach.

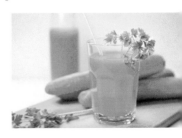

BEET ROOT JUICE

Ingredients

200g/7oz raw beetroot or beets (use fresh beetroot only)

1 carrot

1 large orange

50g/2oz spinach

Step 1

Grab a sharp knife and cut the beetroot into wedges. Chop the carrot roughly then cut away the skin from the orange and roughly slice the flesh.

Step 2

Push the beetroot, orange, and carrot through a juicer, then the spinach last. Pour into a glass and enjoy.

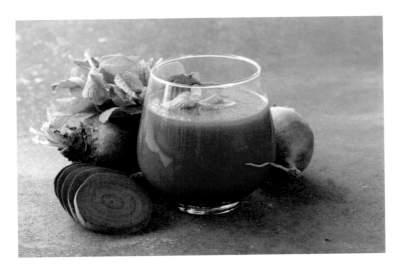

Cucumber - apple juice

INGREDIENTS

1 cucumber
1 green apple (skin on)
1 handful of parsley

Place all ingredients in the juicer, add water if desired, and drink immediately.

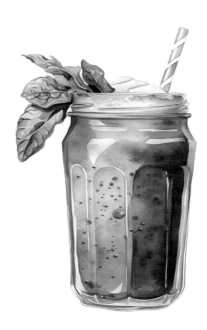

SAMPLE FASTING SCHEDULE:

8:00 AM LEMON WATER

10:00 AM CARROT JUICE

12 NOON BEETROOT JUICE

2:00 PM CUCUMBER APPLE JUICE

4:00 PM VEGETABLE BROTH

6:00 PM CONSUME WATER/LEMON WATER

8:00 PM UNSWEETENED CHAMOMILE,MINT , LEMON BALM OR GREEN TEA

HELPFUL TIPS & STRATEGIES:

DRINK WATER THROUGHOUT THE DAY.

PROTEIN POWDER CAN BE ADDED TO JUICES OR WATER IF HUNGER PERSISTS

1 TSP OF SPIRILINA MAY BE ADDED TO AN 8OZ GLASS OF WATER OR JUICE IF EXPERIENCING LOW BLOOD SUGAR

IF SEVERE HUNGER PERSISTS YOU MAY EAT WATERMELON TO CURB YOUR APPETITE WITHOUT BREAKING THE FAST.

EXTENDING THE PROGRAM

THE 24 HR FAST CAN BE THE BEGINNING OF A DETOX TO LEAD YOU DOWN THE PATH OF A HEALTHY LIFESTYLE CHANGE. THESE CHANGES CAN INCLUDE BUT NOT LIMITED TO:

2 DAY FAST
3 DAY FAST
VEGAN /VEGETARIAN LIFESTYLE
OR CLEAN EATING

MORE MATERIALS TO FOLLOW THANK YOU AGAIN FOR YOUR SUPPORT.

COACH LAWRENCE

EXTENDING THE FAST CONT.

2 DAY FAST

Two-day water/juice fast - After feeling like you have successfully conquered the 24-hour water/juice fast, and feel you are mentally ready to continue. Repeat the 24hr schedule.

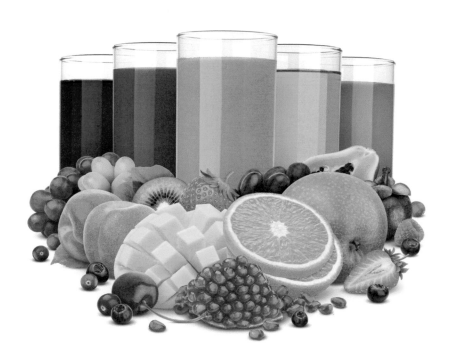

EXTENDING THE PROGRAM CONT:

3 DAY FAST

Three-day water/juice fast - This would be the maximum time I would suggest fasting because at this point your body will have cleansed itself and begun the rejuvenation process.

BREAKING THE FAST: the safest/best way to break the 2 or 3 day fast would be to slowly reintroduce whole fruits and vegetables into your eating regimen.

EXTENDING THE PROGRAM CONT:

VEGAN LIFESTYLE:

<u>Vegan</u> - Consuming only fruits and vegetables, no meat dairy, or eggs.

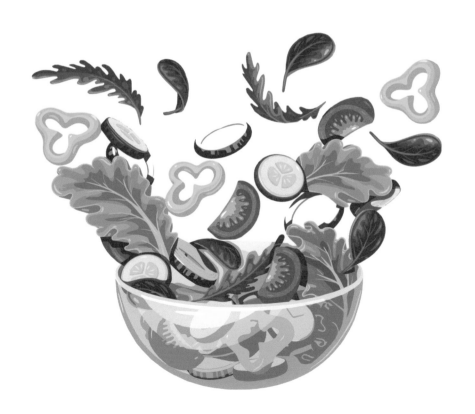

EXTENDING THE PROGRAM CONT:

VEGETARIAN LIFESTYLE:

VEGETARIANISM- Dietary practice of abstaining from meat consumption.

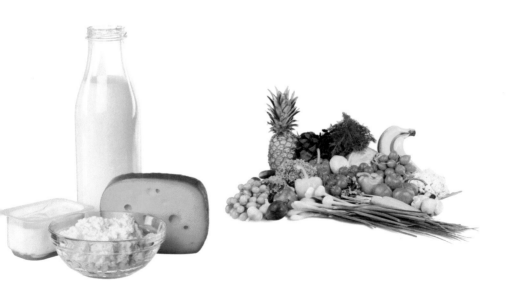

EXTENDING THE PROGRAM CONT:

CLEAN EATING- refers to eating foods that are as close as possible to their natural state. This encourages us to make our meals from scratch to make them as "clean" as possible.

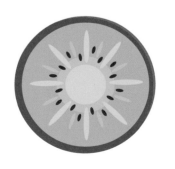
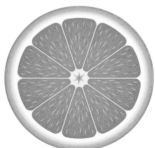
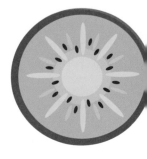

DETERMINATION:

"Determination becomes obsession and then it becomes all that matters"

Jeremy Irvine

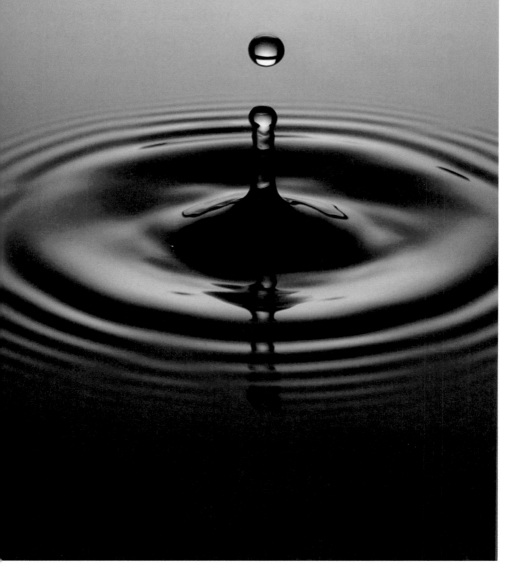

A LITTLE ABOUT COACH LAWRENCE:

I STARTED MY FITNESS JOURNEY AS A PERSONAL TRAINER. IT WAS MY PASSION TO HELP PEOPLE MEET AND EXCEED THEIR FITNESS GOALS. THIS LED ME TO DIVE INTO THE WORLD OF HEALTHY EATING . ON MY PATH TO GAINING MY CERTIFICATION AS A NATURAL HEALTH CONSULTANT IS WHERE I WAS INTRODUCED INTO THE WORLD OF FASTING, VEGANINSM, VEGETARIANISM AND CLEAN EATING. THIS WAS THE FOUNDATION FOR THE REASON BEHIND THE INFORMATION I SHARE WITH YOU IN MY BOOKS TODAY.

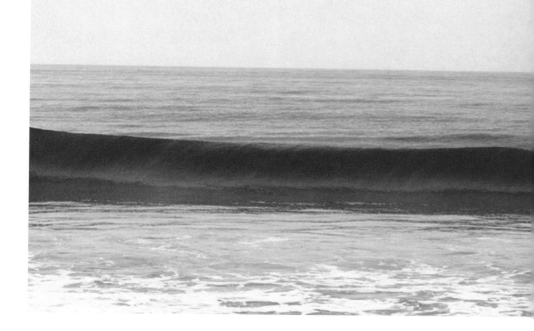

COACH LAWRENCE'S CERTIFICATIONS AND ACCREDITATIONS:

NATURAL HEALTH CONSULTAT/RELAXATION THERAPIST- STRATFORD CAREER INSTITURE

NUTRITIONIST/PERSONAL TRAINER/FITNESS COACH/SPECIALIST IN BODYBUILDING- INT'L SPORTS SCIENCES ASSOCIATION

COLOR THERAPY/PROFESSIONAL RELAXATION THERAPY AND HYPNOTHERAPY- SCHOOL OF NATURAL HEALTH SCIENCES

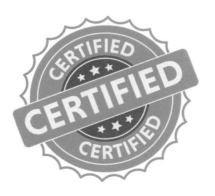

THANK
YOU

Made in United States
Troutdale, OR
06/05/2025

31900802R00017